# Table of Contents

**Introduction** ............................................................. 6
*Importance of healthy eating* ................................................ 7
*Overview of the five methods for optimizing and monitoring eating* ............................................................. 8

**Chapter 1: DNA Nudge** ............................................. 9
*How DNA Nudge works* ....................................................... 9
*Pros of DNA Nudge for healthy eating* ............................ 11
*Cons of DNA Nudge* ............................................................ 14
*Success stories of using DNA Nudge for healthy eating* . 16

**Chapter 2: Food Tracking Apps** ........................... 18
*Overview of popular food tracking apps* ....................... 18
*Benefits of using food tracking apps for healthy eating* .20
*Drawbacks of using food tracking apps* ........................ 22
*Strategies for optimizing food tracking apps for healthy eating* ................................................................. 24

**Chapter 3: Smart Kitchen Appliances** ................ 26
*Overview of smart kitchen appliances for healthy eating* ............................................................................. 26
*Advantages of using smart kitchen appliances* ............ 29
*Drawbacks of using smart kitchen appliances* ............. 31
*Recipes and meal planning strategies for optimizing smart kitchen appliances for healthy eating* ................. 34

**Chapter 4: Nutritional Coaching** ....................... 37

*How nutritional coaching works* ............................ 37
*Benefits of nutritional coaching for healthy eating* ........ 40
*Drawbacks of nutritional coaching* ......................... 42
*Tips for finding and working with a qualified nutritional coach* ............................................. 45

## Chapter 5: Food Sensors .............................. 48
*Overview of food sensors for healthy eating* ............... 48
*Advantages of using food sensors* .......................... 52
*Drawbacks of using food sensors* ........................... 55
*Real-world examples of using food sensors for healthy eating* ..................................................... 58

## Chapter 6: Comparing and Combining Methods ... 61
*Side-by-side comparison of the five methods for optimizing and monitoring eating habits* ................... 61
*Tips for combining methods* ................................ 66
*Real-world examples of using multiple methods for healthy eating" the sub topic for about 3000 words long* ................................................. 69
*Choosing the best methods for your individual needs and preferences* .............................................. 72

## Conclusion ........................................... 75
*Summary of the book's main points* ......................... 75
*Final thoughts on optimizing and monitoring eating habits* .................................................... 78

*Call to action for readers to take control of their health through healthy eating habits*............................................ *81*
**Potential References.................................................84**

## Introduction

Maintaining a healthy diet is an essential aspect of a healthy lifestyle. Eating a balanced diet can help prevent a range of chronic diseases, such as heart disease, diabetes, and cancer, and can also improve mental health, boost energy levels, and support a healthy weight. Despite the known benefits of healthy eating, however, many people struggle to maintain a healthy diet in the face of busy schedules, unhealthy food options, and conflicting nutritional advice.

## Importance of healthy eating

This section will explore the importance of healthy eating in greater detail, highlighting the various benefits of maintaining a healthy diet. We will begin by examining the relationship between nutrition and overall health, exploring the role of nutrients in supporting various bodily systems and functions. We will also discuss the link between healthy eating and disease prevention, highlighting the role of a healthy diet in reducing the risk of chronic diseases.

In addition, this section will explore the impact of healthy eating on mental health and wellbeing, highlighting the ways in which a healthy diet can support cognitive function and emotional regulation. We will also discuss the role of healthy eating in maintaining a healthy weight, exploring the link between nutrition and metabolism.

Overall, this section will provide a comprehensive overview of the importance of healthy eating, emphasizing the numerous benefits of maintaining a healthy diet and the impact that nutrition can have on overall health and wellbeing. By setting the stage for the rest of the book, this section will help readers understand the importance of optimizing and monitoring their eating habits to support their long-term health goals.

## Overview of the five methods for optimizing and monitoring eating

In this section of the introduction, we will provide an overview of the five methods for optimizing and monitoring eating habits that will be discussed in the following chapters. The aim of this section is to give readers an understanding of the different approaches available to them for improving their eating habits and making healthier choices.

We will discuss the five methods in brief, including their unique features, benefits, and potential drawbacks. This will include a high-level overview of how DNA Nudge works, the advantages of using food tracking apps, the benefits of using smart kitchen appliances, the advantages of nutritional coaching, and the ways in which food sensors can help with healthy eating.

By providing a comprehensive overview of these methods, we hope to give readers a clear understanding of the options available to them and to help them choose the most effective method or combination of methods for their individual needs and preferences. We will also highlight the importance of monitoring eating habits and the potential benefits of doing so, such as improved weight management, increased energy levels, and reduced risk of chronic diseases.

# Chapter 1: DNA Nudge

## How DNA Nudge works

DNA Nudge is a personalized nutrition and lifestyle program that uses genetic testing to help individuals optimize their eating habits. The process begins with a simple DNA test, which analyzes an individual's unique genetic code to determine how their body processes different nutrients.

The DNA Nudge program provides users with a wrist-worn device called the DNA Band, which acts as a personalized nutrition coach. The DNA Band uses the results of the genetic test to guide users towards healthy food choices by scanning barcodes of food products and providing a green or red light based on whether the food is a good match for the user's genetic profile.

The DNA Nudge program also includes an app that provides users with personalized nutrition plans, shopping lists, and recipe suggestions based on their genetic profile. The app also tracks physical activity and sleep, which are important factors in overall health and wellbeing.

The genetic testing process used by DNA Nudge is based on years of research into the relationship between genetics and nutrition. The company uses a proprietary algorithm to analyze an individual's genetic data and provide personalized nutrition recommendations. The genetic testing is done using a simple saliva sample, which can be collected at home and sent back to the company for analysis.

Overall, the DNA Nudge program is designed to help individuals make informed choices about their diet and lifestyle based on their unique genetic makeup. By understanding how their body processes different nutrients, users can make more effective choices about what to eat and when, which can lead to improved health outcomes over time.

## Pros of DNA Nudge for healthy eating

DNA Nudge is a unique and innovative method for optimizing and monitoring eating habits. By analyzing an individual's DNA, the system can provide personalized nutritional recommendations and help individuals make healthier food choices. There are several advantages of using DNA Nudge for healthy eating, including:

1. Personalized Recommendations: The most significant advantage of DNA Nudge is that it provides personalized nutritional recommendations. Based on an individual's DNA analysis, the system can identify which foods are best suited for their body, and which foods they should avoid. This level of personalization is impossible to achieve with other methods, such as food tracking apps or smart kitchen appliances.

2. Science-Backed: DNA Nudge is based on scientific research and has been shown to be effective in improving eating habits. The system was developed by Imperial College London, and its efficacy has been demonstrated in several clinical trials. This scientific backing gives individuals the confidence that the recommendations provided by the system are evidence-based and have a solid scientific foundation.

3. User-Friendly: DNA Nudge is user-friendly and easy to use. Individuals can use a wearable device that scans the barcode of food products, and the system will provide instant recommendations based on their DNA. The system also provides an app that can be used to track progress and monitor nutritional intake. The app is intuitive and easy to use, making it an attractive option for individuals who want to make healthier food choices but may not have the time or energy to track their food intake manually.

4. Long-Term Benefits: DNA Nudge is designed to provide long-term benefits for healthy eating. By providing personalized recommendations based on an individual's DNA, the system can help individuals make sustainable changes to their diet that can lead to long-term health benefits. The system encourages individuals to make healthier food choices, which can lead to weight loss, improved gut health, and reduced risk of chronic diseases such as diabetes and heart disease.

Overall, DNA Nudge is a promising method for optimizing and monitoring eating habits. It provides personalized recommendations based on an individual's DNA, is science-backed, user-friendly, and provides long-term benefits for healthy eating. While there are some drawbacks to using DNA Nudge, such as the cost and the need for DNA analysis, the system's advantages make it an attractive option for individuals who want to make sustainable changes to their diet and improve their health.

## Cons of DNA Nudge

While DNA Nudge can be a powerful tool for optimizing and monitoring healthy eating habits, it is not without its drawbacks. Some of the potential downsides of DNA Nudge include:

1. Cost: The DNA Nudge system can be expensive, with a one-time cost of several hundred dollars for the initial test and ongoing costs for the app and additional sensors.

2. Limited food database: The DNA Nudge system relies on a database of foods and ingredients to make recommendations, and this database may not be comprehensive enough to include all the foods an individual may consume. This can result in inaccurate or incomplete recommendations.

3. Privacy concerns: Some individuals may be hesitant to share their genetic information with a third-party company, even one that claims to use it for health purposes. Additionally, the data collected by DNA Nudge could potentially be accessed or used by unauthorized parties, which raises concerns about data privacy and security.

4. Limited focus on other health factors: While DNA Nudge can provide insight into an individual's genetic predispositions and food sensitivities, it may not take into account other important factors such as physical activity,

sleep, stress, and overall medical history. This means that the system may not provide a comprehensive or personalized approach to healthy eating.

5. Limited efficacy: While some individuals may see significant improvements in their eating habits using DNA Nudge, others may not experience as much benefit. Additionally, DNA Nudge may not be effective for all types of individuals, such as those with complex medical conditions or food allergies.

It's important to carefully consider these potential drawbacks before deciding whether to use DNA Nudge for optimizing and monitoring healthy eating habits. It may be worth weighing the pros and cons and exploring other methods to find the most effective approach for your individual needs and preferences.

## Success stories of using DNA Nudge for healthy eating

DNA Nudge is a relatively new technology, but it has already shown promising results in helping individuals make healthier food choices. In this section, we will explore some success stories of people who have used DNA Nudge to improve their eating habits and overall health.

One success story is that of Sarah, a busy mother of three who had struggled to lose weight and maintain a healthy diet for years. Despite her best efforts, she found herself constantly reaching for sugary snacks and high-calorie meals. After taking the DNA Nudge test, she discovered that she had a genetic predisposition to weight gain and a sensitivity to sugar. With this knowledge, she was able to make more informed food choices and was even able to use the DNA Nudge wristband to receive real-time recommendations on what to eat while out and about.

Another success story is that of John, a middle-aged man who had a family history of heart disease and high blood pressure. After taking the DNA Nudge test, he learned that he had a higher-than-average risk for developing these conditions. With this knowledge, he was motivated to make healthier food choices and was able to use the DNA Nudge app to track his progress and receive personalized food recommendations.

Overall, these success stories demonstrate the potential of DNA Nudge to help individuals make healthier food choices and improve their overall health. While the technology is still in its early stages, the results are promising, and many individuals have already seen significant improvements in their eating habits and health outcomes.

## Chapter 2: Food Tracking Apps
### Overview of popular food tracking apps

There are many food tracking apps available for users to download and use, and each app has its unique features and benefits. Here are some of the most popular food tracking apps that users can consider using:

1. MyFitnessPal: MyFitnessPal is one of the most popular food tracking apps, with over 200 million users worldwide. It allows users to track their calorie intake, nutrient intake, and exercise. The app offers a comprehensive food database and barcode scanner for easy tracking, and it also has a feature for tracking water intake.

2. Lose It!: Lose It! is another popular food tracking app that offers similar features to MyFitnessPal. It also has a comprehensive food database, barcode scanner, and the ability to track nutrient intake. One unique feature of Lose It! is its ability to connect with various fitness trackers and smart scales.

3. Lifesum: Lifesum is a food tracking app that offers a more holistic approach to healthy eating. In addition to tracking calorie and nutrient intake, it offers personalized meal plans and recipes, water and step tracking, and a variety of diets to choose from.

4. FatSecret: FatSecret is a free food tracking app that offers similar features to other food tracking apps. However, it also offers a community aspect where users can connect with each other, share recipes, and offer support.

5. SparkPeople: SparkPeople is a food tracking app that offers a comprehensive database of over 4 million foods. It also offers a community aspect where users can connect with each other, share recipes, and offer support.

These are just a few of the most popular food tracking apps, but there are many more available for users to choose from. It's important to consider the features and benefits of each app to find the one that best suits your needs and preferences.

## Benefits of using food tracking apps for healthy eating

Food tracking apps are designed to help users monitor their food intake, making them an excellent tool for promoting healthy eating. Here are some of the benefits of using food tracking apps:

1. Increases awareness of food intake: Food tracking apps allow users to input the food they eat, which helps them keep track of their calorie intake and nutritional information. This can increase their awareness of what they're eating, making them more mindful of their food choices.

2. Helps with portion control: Many food tracking apps allow users to track portion sizes, making it easier for them to control their food intake. This is particularly helpful for individuals trying to lose weight or maintain a healthy weight.

3. Encourages healthier food choices: Food tracking apps often provide users with nutritional information, including calories, macronutrients, and micronutrients. This can help users make more informed food choices and opt for healthier options.

4. Provides accountability: Food tracking apps can help users stay accountable for their food choices. Knowing that they have to input their food intake into the app can

motivate them to make healthier choices and avoid overeating.

5. Customizable goals: Many food tracking apps allow users to set personalized goals, such as daily calorie intake or macronutrient ratios. This can help users stay motivated and focused on their healthy eating goals.

Overall, food tracking apps can be a valuable tool for promoting healthy eating. By increasing awareness, encouraging healthier choices, and providing accountability, they can help individuals achieve their health and fitness goals.

## Drawbacks of using food tracking apps

Food tracking apps have become increasingly popular in recent years as people become more health-conscious and strive to achieve their fitness and nutrition goals. While food tracking apps can be extremely useful tools for healthy eating, there are also several drawbacks to consider.

1. Time-consuming and tedious One of the most significant drawbacks of food tracking apps is that they can be time-consuming and tedious to use. To be effective, these apps require users to enter every food and drink they consume, including portion sizes and macronutrient breakdowns. This process can be time-consuming and require a significant amount of effort to keep up with consistently.

2. Inaccuracy Another drawback of food tracking apps is the potential for inaccuracy. These apps rely on user input, and there is always the risk of error when it comes to estimating portion sizes or macronutrient content. Additionally, many apps rely on crowdsourced data for their nutrition information, which can be inaccurate or incomplete.

3. Can be triggering for those with eating disorders Food tracking apps can also be triggering for individuals with a history of disordered eating or eating disorders. Tracking

every calorie and macro can quickly become obsessive and compulsive, leading to an unhealthy fixation on food and potential relapse.

4. Doesn't necessarily promote intuitive eating Some experts argue that food tracking apps can actually detract from the practice of intuitive eating. By relying on an app to tell you what to eat, rather than listening to your body's natural hunger and fullness cues, you may be less in tune with your body's needs and more likely to develop an unhealthy relationship with food.

5. Can be expensive While many food tracking apps are free to download, some of the more advanced features may require a subscription or payment. This can be a financial barrier for some individuals, making it difficult to fully utilize the app's features.

Overall, while food tracking apps can be beneficial for those looking to improve their nutrition and overall health, it's essential to consider the potential drawbacks before deciding to use one. It's important to approach these apps with a balanced perspective and not rely on them as the sole source of nutritional guidance.

## Strategies for optimizing food tracking apps for healthy eating

Food tracking apps can be a valuable tool for anyone looking to improve their eating habits. However, like any tool, they can be used more effectively with the right strategies. Here are some strategies for optimizing food tracking apps for healthy eating:

1. Set specific goals: Before using a food tracking app, it's important to set specific goals. These goals can be anything from losing weight to improving overall nutrition. By setting clear goals, users can tailor their food tracking to their specific needs.

2. Be consistent: For a food tracking app to be effective, users need to be consistent in tracking their meals. This means tracking everything they eat, including snacks and drinks. Consistency is key when it comes to using a food tracking app.

3. Customize the app: Most food tracking apps allow users to customize the app to their needs. This might include setting reminders to log meals or customizing the app to track specific nutrients. By customizing the app, users can make it more effective for their specific goals.

4. Use the barcode scanner: Many food tracking apps include a barcode scanner that allows users to quickly and

easily log their meals. This can be a great way to save time and ensure that all meals are tracked accurately.

5. Plan meals in advance: Planning meals in advance can make it easier to track meals using a food tracking app. By planning meals in advance, users can ensure that they have healthy options available and can easily log their meals in the app.

6. Use the app's social features: Many food tracking apps include social features that allow users to connect with others who are also using the app. This can be a great way to stay motivated and get support from others who are working towards similar goals.

7. Be mindful of portion sizes: While food tracking apps can be helpful for tracking nutrients, they don't always account for portion sizes. Users should be mindful of portion sizes when tracking meals and make adjustments as needed to ensure they're meeting their goals.

By using these strategies, users can optimize their food tracking apps for healthy eating and get the most out of this valuable tool.

## Chapter 3: Smart Kitchen Appliances
### Overview of smart kitchen appliances for healthy eating

Smart kitchen appliances are becoming increasingly popular in modern homes due to the convenience and efficiency they offer. These appliances can be connected to the internet and controlled through smartphone apps or voice assistants, making cooking and meal preparation more accessible and manageable for people with busy lifestyles. Smart kitchen appliances can also help to promote healthy eating habits by providing features and functions that make it easier to prepare healthy meals at home.

Here are some of the most popular types of smart kitchen appliances that can be used to support healthy eating:

1. Smart Refrigerators Smart refrigerators can help you keep track of the food in your fridge and provide suggestions for meals based on the ingredients you have on hand. Some models can even keep track of expiration dates and alert you when it's time to use up certain foods before they go bad. This can help you reduce food waste and ensure that you always have fresh ingredients on hand for healthy meals.

2. Smart Ovens Smart ovens can be programmed to cook your meals perfectly every time, with options for baking, roasting, broiling, and more. Some models also come with features like steam cooking, which can help to preserve the nutrients in your food. Additionally, some smart ovens have cameras that allow you to monitor your food as it cooks from your smartphone.

3. Smart Cooktops Smart cooktops can be programmed to cook your food to the exact temperature you want, which can be important for maintaining the nutrient content of your food. Some models also have built-in sensors that can detect the size of your cookware and adjust the heat accordingly to ensure even cooking.

4. Smart Blenders Smart blenders can make it easy to whip up healthy smoothies and other blended recipes. Some models can connect to your smartphone and provide recipes and suggestions for healthy smoothie combinations based on your dietary preferences.

5. Smart Coffee Makers Smart coffee makers can be programmed to brew your coffee at specific times, and some models also allow you to customize your coffee's strength and flavor. This can help you avoid buying expensive coffee drinks at coffee shops and ensure that you're starting your day with a healthy and energizing beverage.

Overall, smart kitchen appliances can make it easier and more convenient to prepare healthy meals at home. By taking advantage of the features and functions of these appliances, you can ensure that you're eating nutritious meals that support your health and wellbeing.

### Advantages of using smart kitchen appliances

Smart kitchen appliances are becoming increasingly popular due to the convenience they offer. These appliances can be programmed to perform specific tasks, such as cooking or blending, at specific times, making it easier to stick to a healthy eating plan. Some of the advantages of using smart kitchen appliances for healthy eating include:

1. Saves time: Smart kitchen appliances can save time when preparing meals. For example, a smart blender can quickly make a smoothie, and a smart cooker can prepare a healthy meal while you attend to other tasks.

2. More accurate portion control: Smart kitchen appliances can help with portion control. For example, a smart scale can weigh ingredients, making it easier to accurately measure portion sizes.

3. Reduces food waste: Smart kitchen appliances can help reduce food waste by keeping track of expiration dates and notifying the user when food needs to be used.

4. Encourages healthy habits: Smart kitchen appliances can help users develop healthy habits by providing them with healthy recipes and ingredient suggestions.

5. Customizable settings: Smart kitchen appliances can be programmed to meet individual needs. For example, a

smart oven can be set to cook meals according to individual preferences, such as cooking time and temperature.

6. Offers remote control: Many smart kitchen appliances can be controlled remotely, making it possible to start cooking while away from home. This can be especially useful for people who work long hours or have busy schedules.

7. Provides nutritional information: Some smart kitchen appliances, such as smart scales and smart blenders, can provide nutritional information for the foods they prepare. This can be helpful for people who are tracking their calorie intake or are trying to follow a specific diet.

Overall, using smart kitchen appliances can provide several advantages for healthy eating, including time savings, accurate portion control, and the ability to develop healthy habits. By taking advantage of these benefits, individuals can make healthy eating more convenient and enjoyable.

## Drawbacks of using smart kitchen appliances

Smart kitchen appliances have the potential to make healthy eating easier and more convenient, but they are not without their drawbacks. Here are some of the main drawbacks to consider:

1. Cost: One of the biggest drawbacks to smart kitchen appliances is their cost. They can be significantly more expensive than traditional appliances, which may not be feasible for everyone. Additionally, some smart kitchen appliances require additional components, such as special cookware or sensors, that can add to the cost.

2. Technical issues: As with any technology, smart kitchen appliances can experience technical issues that may require professional repairs. If a smart appliance malfunctions, it may not be possible to use it until the issue is resolved, which can be frustrating and time-consuming.

3. Limited functionality: While smart kitchen appliances can offer a wide range of features, not all appliances are created equal. Some may have limited functionality or be less intuitive to use than others. This can be particularly problematic for those who are not particularly tech-savvy or who are trying to balance multiple tasks in the kitchen.

4. Reliance on technology: Smart kitchen appliances are heavily reliant on technology, and may not be as useful if the technology fails. This can be particularly problematic during power outages or if there are issues with the Wi-Fi or other connected devices.

5. Privacy concerns: Smart kitchen appliances often collect data about usage patterns and other personal information, which can raise privacy concerns for some users. While some manufacturers may have policies in place to protect user data, it's important to read the fine print and understand how your data is being used.

6. Lack of flexibility: While smart kitchen appliances can make it easier to cook healthy meals, they may also limit flexibility in some ways. For example, some smart ovens may not allow users to adjust the temperature or cooking time manually, which can be frustrating for more experienced cooks.

7. Learning curve: Using smart kitchen appliances may require a learning curve, as users adjust to new features and functionality. This can be particularly challenging for older adults or those with limited experience using technology.

While there are some drawbacks to using smart kitchen appliances, many people find that the benefits outweigh the challenges. It's important to weigh the pros and cons carefully and choose the right appliance based on your needs and budget.

## Recipes and meal planning strategies for optimizing smart kitchen appliances for healthy eating

Smart kitchen appliances can be a valuable tool for optimizing healthy eating. However, to get the most out of these appliances, it's important to use them in conjunction with effective recipes and meal planning strategies. Here are some tips for using smart kitchen appliances to optimize healthy eating:

1. Meal Planning: Planning is key to healthy eating, and it's even more important when using smart kitchen appliances. Before you start cooking, plan out what you're going to make and how you'll use the appliance. Consider factors like cooking time, temperature, and portion size to make sure you get the most out of your appliance.

2. Use Healthy Recipes: There are countless recipes available online and in cookbooks that are specifically designed for smart kitchen appliances. When choosing a recipe, look for one that's high in nutrients and fits your dietary goals. There are many websites and apps available that provide healthy recipes for smart kitchen appliances.

3. Cook Ahead: Smart kitchen appliances can be used to make meal prep easier, and can be a great tool for cooking ahead. Consider using the slow cooker, pressure cooker, or air fryer to make large batches of meals that can be portioned

out and eaten throughout the week. This can save time and make it easier to stick to a healthy eating plan.

4. Experiment with Different Ingredients: Smart kitchen appliances can be used to cook a variety of different ingredients, from vegetables to meats and grains. Experiment with different ingredients and recipes to find what works best for you. Consider using ingredients that are in season, or that are locally sourced, to get the freshest and most nutritious foods possible.

5. Monitor Portion Sizes: Smart kitchen appliances can be great for portion control, but it's important to make sure you're monitoring portion sizes. Use a food scale or measuring cups to make sure you're eating the right amount of food. Overeating, even with healthy foods, can lead to weight gain and other health problems.

6. Consider Your Specific Needs: When using smart kitchen appliances, it's important to consider your specific dietary needs. For example, if you're following a low-carb diet, you may want to look for recipes that are high in protein and healthy fats. If you're vegetarian or vegan, you'll want to focus on recipes that are high in plant-based protein.

7. Get Creative: Finally, don't be afraid to get creative with your smart kitchen appliances. Try new recipes, experiment with different ingredients, and have fun. Smart

kitchen appliances can be a great way to explore new foods and cooking methods, and can be a valuable tool for optimizing healthy eating.

## Chapter 4: Nutritional Coaching
## How nutritional coaching works

Nutritional coaching is a form of personalized support and guidance for individuals who are seeking to improve their eating habits and achieve better health outcomes. Nutritional coaches are trained professionals who specialize in nutrition and wellness, and they work with their clients to develop individualized nutrition plans and provide ongoing support and accountability.

Nutritional coaching typically begins with an initial consultation, during which the coach will gather information about the client's health history, dietary habits, and lifestyle. Based on this information, the coach will develop a personalized nutrition plan that takes into account the client's individual needs, preferences, and goals.

The nutrition plan may include recommendations for specific foods and nutrients, as well as guidance on portion sizes and meal timing. The coach may also provide tips and strategies for making healthy choices when eating out, grocery shopping, and cooking at home.

Throughout the coaching process, the coach will work with the client to monitor their progress and make adjustments to the nutrition plan as needed. The coach may also provide ongoing support and accountability, such as regular check-ins and tracking of food intake and physical activity.

One of the key benefits of nutritional coaching is the personalized and individualized approach to nutrition. Unlike generic diet plans or fad diets, nutritional coaching takes into account the unique needs and circumstances of each individual client. This can lead to better outcomes and more sustainable changes in eating habits.

Nutritional coaching may also provide education and information about nutrition and health, helping clients to better understand the impact of their food choices on their overall well-being. This can help to empower clients to make informed decisions about their health and nutrition.

Another potential benefit of nutritional coaching is the accountability and support that it provides. Many people struggle to make healthy changes on their own, and having the support and guidance of a coach can make a significant difference. Coaches can help to identify obstacles and provide strategies for overcoming them, as well as offer encouragement and motivation throughout the process.

However, it is important to note that nutritional coaching may not be suitable or effective for everyone. People with certain health conditions or dietary restrictions may require specialized care from a registered dietitian or healthcare provider. Additionally, nutritional coaching may be expensive and may not be covered by insurance.

In summary, nutritional coaching is a personalized and individualized approach to nutrition that can provide support, guidance, and accountability for individuals seeking to improve their eating habits and achieve better health outcomes. By working with a trained nutritional coach, clients can develop a tailored nutrition plan that takes into account their unique needs, preferences, and goals, and receive ongoing support and monitoring throughout the process. While nutritional coaching may not be suitable or effective for everyone, it can be a valuable tool for those looking to make sustainable and meaningful changes in their eating habits and overall health.

## Benefits of nutritional coaching for healthy eating

Nutritional coaching involves working with a registered dietitian or nutritionist who provides personalized guidance and support to help individuals improve their eating habits and overall health. Here are some benefits of nutritional coaching for healthy eating:

1. Personalized guidance: Nutritional coaching provides personalized guidance based on an individual's unique needs, preferences, and goals. A registered dietitian or nutritionist can develop a customized meal plan and offer tailored recommendations for healthy eating, taking into account factors such as dietary restrictions, food preferences, and lifestyle habits.

2. Improved eating habits: Nutritional coaching can help individuals develop better eating habits, such as eating more fruits and vegetables, reducing sugar and salt intake, and choosing whole, minimally processed foods. With the help of a coach, individuals can learn to make healthier choices and develop a sustainable approach to healthy eating.

3. Disease prevention and management: Nutritional coaching can help individuals prevent or manage chronic diseases such as diabetes, heart disease, and obesity. A registered dietitian or nutritionist can provide education on

how certain foods and nutrients impact health and offer specific recommendations to support disease prevention or management.

4. Accountability and support: Nutritional coaching provides accountability and support to help individuals stay on track with their healthy eating goals. Coaches can help clients identify and overcome barriers to healthy eating, provide motivation and encouragement, and offer practical strategies for making healthy eating a sustainable habit.

5. Long-term success: Nutritional coaching can provide individuals with the knowledge and skills needed to make lasting changes to their eating habits. By working with a coach, individuals can develop a personalized plan for healthy eating that is tailored to their needs and preferences, and that can be sustained over the long term.

Overall, nutritional coaching can be a valuable tool for improving eating habits and overall health. By working with a registered dietitian or nutritionist, individuals can receive personalized guidance and support to develop sustainable healthy eating habits that can last a lifetime.

## Drawbacks of nutritional coaching

Nutritional coaching has several benefits for individuals seeking to improve their eating habits and overall health. However, there are also some drawbacks that should be considered before deciding to pursue this option.

One of the main drawbacks of nutritional coaching is the cost. Nutritional coaching sessions can be expensive, and some people may not be able to afford them. Additionally, some insurance plans do not cover the cost of nutritional coaching, which can make it even more difficult for some people to access this service.

Another potential drawback is that nutritional coaching can be time-consuming. It requires a commitment to attending regular coaching sessions and following through on the recommendations made by the coach. For some people, this may be a significant barrier to accessing nutritional coaching.

In addition, not all nutritional coaches are created equal. While some coaches are highly qualified and experienced, others may lack the necessary credentials and expertise to provide effective coaching. This can make it difficult for individuals to find a coach who is a good fit for their needs and who can provide the level of support they require.

Finally, nutritional coaching may not be suitable for everyone. People who have complex medical conditions or who are taking certain medications may require more specialized guidance than can be provided by a general nutritional coach. In these cases, it may be necessary to work with a registered dietitian or other healthcare provider who can provide more targeted guidance.

Despite these drawbacks, there are many benefits to working with a nutritional coach. For individuals who are committed to making positive changes to their eating habits, a coach can provide valuable guidance and support. Some of the benefits of nutritional coaching include:

1. Personalized guidance: A nutritional coach can work with clients to develop a customized eating plan that takes into account their unique goals, preferences, and dietary needs. This can help ensure that individuals are making the most of their meals and are getting the nutrients they need to support their health.

2. Accountability: Nutritional coaching provides a level of accountability that can be difficult to achieve on one's own. Knowing that they will be reporting back to their coach can help individuals stay on track with their healthy eating goals.

3. Education: Nutritional coaches can provide clients with the information they need to make informed choices about their diet. This can include information about the nutritional value of different foods, the impact of certain dietary choices on health, and strategies for making healthy choices when eating out or traveling.

4. Motivation: Nutritional coaching can help individuals stay motivated and focused on their goals. Coaches can provide encouragement and support, helping individuals to overcome challenges and stay on track with their healthy eating habits.

5. Long-term success: Working with a nutritional coach can provide individuals with the skills and knowledge they need to make lasting changes to their eating habits. This can help promote long-term success in achieving and maintaining a healthy weight, improving overall health, and reducing the risk of chronic disease.

In conclusion, while there are some drawbacks to nutritional coaching, the benefits can make it a valuable tool for individuals seeking to improve their eating habits and overall health. By providing personalized guidance, accountability, education, motivation, and long-term success, nutritional coaching can be an effective way to achieve and maintain healthy eating habits.

## Tips for finding and working with a qualified nutritional coach

Nutritional coaching is a powerful tool for those seeking to improve their overall health and well-being through healthy eating habits. However, it can be challenging to know how to find a qualified and reputable nutritional coach. In this section, we will discuss some tips for finding and working with a qualified nutritional coach.

1. Look for Accreditation: The first and most crucial step when looking for a nutritional coach is to ensure that they are accredited by a reputable organization such as the International Coach Federation (ICF) or the National Board for Health and Wellness Coaching (NBHWC). Accreditation ensures that the coach has undergone rigorous training and has the necessary skills and experience to provide effective nutritional coaching.

2. Consider Their Area of Expertise: There are several different types of nutritional coaches, and they may have different areas of expertise, such as sports nutrition, weight loss, or disease prevention. It is essential to find a coach whose expertise aligns with your health goals and needs.

3. Look for Reviews and Testimonials: Reading reviews and testimonials from previous clients is an excellent way to gauge a coach's effectiveness and determine if they

are a good fit for you. Look for coaches with a proven track record of success and positive feedback from their clients.

4. Evaluate Their Approach: Nutritional coaching approaches can vary widely, from a holistic approach to a more structured approach. It is essential to choose a coach whose approach aligns with your personality and learning style. Some coaches may be more focused on behavior modification, while others may take a more educational approach.

5. Consider Their Availability: Some coaches may have a limited availability, and others may be more flexible. Consider your schedule and availability when choosing a coach to ensure that their availability aligns with your needs.

6. Determine Their Cost: The cost of nutritional coaching can vary widely, depending on the coach's qualifications, location, and experience. It is essential to determine the coach's cost upfront to ensure that it aligns with your budget.

7. Be Open and Honest: Once you have found a coach that aligns with your needs and goals, it is essential to be open and honest during your coaching sessions. Nutritional coaches can only provide effective coaching when they have a clear understanding of your health goals, needs, and challenges.

In conclusion, finding a qualified and reputable nutritional coach requires some research and due diligence. However, working with a qualified coach can be a powerful tool for those seeking to improve their health through healthy eating habits. By following the tips above, you can find a coach that aligns with your needs and provides the support and guidance you need to achieve your health goals.

## Chapter 5: Food Sensors

## Overview of food sensors for healthy eating

Food sensors are devices that can analyze and provide information about the food we consume. These sensors come in various forms and use different technologies to collect and transmit data. In this chapter, we will provide an overview of food sensors and how they can be used to support healthy eating.

1. Types of Food Sensors There are different types of food sensors, including:

- RFID (Radio-Frequency Identification) Tags: These are small electronic devices that can be attached to food packaging to track and monitor the food's movement through the supply chain. RFID tags can provide information about the food's origin, storage conditions, and expiration date.

- Spectroscopy: Spectroscopy is a technique that uses light to measure the properties of matter. Food sensors that use spectroscopy can analyze the composition of food and provide information about its nutritional content.

- Electrochemical Sensors: These sensors use electrical signals to detect the presence of certain molecules in food. Electrochemical sensors can be used to monitor food quality and detect harmful contaminants.

- Gas Sensors: Gas sensors can detect the presence of gases that are released by food as it spoils. These sensors can be used to monitor the freshness of food and help prevent food waste.

2. Advantages of Food Sensors Food sensors offer several advantages for healthy eating, including:

- Accurate Nutritional Information: Food sensors can provide accurate information about the nutritional content of food, including its calorie, fat, and sugar content. This information can help people make informed choices about what they eat and support healthy eating habits.

- Improved Food Safety: Food sensors can detect harmful contaminants and pathogens in food, helping to prevent foodborne illness. This can be especially important for people with weakened immune systems or those who are at risk for foodborne illnesses.

- Reduced Food Waste: Food sensors can help reduce food waste by providing information about the freshness and quality of food. This can help people make better decisions about when to consume or discard food, reducing the amount of food that goes to waste.

3. Drawbacks of Food Sensors Despite the advantages, there are also some drawbacks to using food sensors, including:

- Cost: Some food sensors can be expensive, which may make them inaccessible to some people.

- Complexity: Some food sensors may require specialized knowledge or training to use and interpret the data they provide.

- Limited Availability: Currently, not all types of food sensors are widely available or accessible to the general public.

4. Examples of Food Sensors There are several food sensors currently available or in development, including:

- SCiO: A handheld spectrometer that can scan food and provide information about its nutritional content.

- Tellspec: A sensor that can be attached to a smartphone to analyze the composition of food and provide information about its nutritional content.

- Kavosmart: A wearable sensor that can monitor the wearer's food intake and provide feedback on their eating habits.

1. Conclusion Food sensors offer a promising way to support healthy eating by providing accurate information about the nutritional content of food, improving food safety, and reducing food waste. However, there are also some drawbacks to consider, including cost and limited availability. As the technology continues to develop, food

sensors have the potential to play an increasingly important role in supporting healthy eating habits.

## Advantages of using food sensors

Food sensors have emerged as a new technology that can help people make healthier food choices by providing accurate information about the nutrient content of their food. There are several advantages to using food sensors for healthy eating.

1. Accurate Nutrient Information: One of the main advantages of using food sensors is that they provide accurate information about the nutrient content of the food you are eating. This information can help you make more informed choices about what to eat and how much to eat. Food sensors use a variety of methods to detect and analyze the nutrient content of food, including spectrometry, electrochemistry, and impedance. Some sensors can detect specific nutrients, such as glucose or sodium, while others can provide a more comprehensive analysis of multiple nutrients.

2. Personalization: Food sensors can also provide personalized information about the nutrient content of your food. Some sensors can be linked to mobile apps that provide real-time feedback about your nutrient intake and suggest personalized recommendations for healthier eating. This personalization can help you identify patterns in your eating habits and make adjustments to your diet accordingly.

3. Convenience: Food sensors are typically small and portable, making them easy to use in a variety of settings. Some sensors are designed to be worn as a device, such as a wristband or necklace, while others can be placed directly on the food. This convenience makes it easier to track your nutrient intake throughout the day, even when you are on the go.

4. Improved Health Outcomes: Using food sensors can also lead to improved health outcomes. By providing more accurate information about the nutrient content of your food, you can make more informed choices about what to eat and how much to eat. This can lead to improved blood sugar control, lower blood pressure, and improved cholesterol levels, among other health benefits.

5. Greater Transparency: Food sensors can also provide greater transparency about the food you are eating. This can be especially useful for people with food allergies or intolerances, as well as those who are concerned about the use of additives or preservatives in their food. By providing more detailed information about the food you are eating, food sensors can help you make more informed choices about what to eat.

Overall, using food sensors can be a valuable tool for healthy eating. By providing more accurate and personalized information about the nutrient content of your food, food sensors can help you make more informed choices about what to eat and how much to eat, leading to improved health outcomes.

## Drawbacks of using food sensors

Food sensors are becoming increasingly popular as a way to monitor food intake and help people make healthier choices. However, like any new technology, they have some drawbacks. In this section, we will explore some of the potential downsides of using food sensors.

1. Cost Food sensors can be expensive, and the price may be prohibitive for some people. While the cost of food sensors has decreased in recent years, they can still be pricey, especially for high-end models that offer more advanced features. This may make them less accessible to people who are on a tight budget.

2. Limited Accuracy Although food sensors are becoming more accurate, they are not yet perfect. They may not be able to differentiate between foods that look similar, and they may not be able to accurately measure the exact amount of a particular nutrient in a food. This means that people who rely solely on food sensors to monitor their nutrient intake may not be getting an accurate picture of what they are consuming.

3. Inconvenience Using food sensors can be time-consuming and inconvenient. People may have to stop what they are doing to take a reading or scan a barcode, which can be frustrating, especially if they are in a rush. Additionally,

food sensors may not be suitable for use in all settings, such as when dining out or at social events.

4. Need for Frequent Calibration Food sensors need to be calibrated regularly to ensure that they are providing accurate readings. This can be time-consuming and may require the use of additional equipment. If food sensors are not calibrated frequently, they may provide inaccurate readings, which can lead to poor dietary choices.

5. Dependence on Technology People who rely heavily on food sensors may become overly dependent on technology to make dietary choices. While food sensors can be a helpful tool, they should not be the sole means of monitoring food intake. People should also be able to make informed dietary choices based on their own knowledge and understanding of nutrition.

6. Potential for Obsessive Behavior Some people may become obsessed with using food sensors to monitor their nutrient intake. This can lead to an unhealthy fixation on food and may even lead to disordered eating behaviors. It is important to use food sensors in moderation and to maintain a healthy perspective on nutrition and dietary choices.

7. Lack of Personalization While food sensors can provide valuable data about nutrient intake, they may not take into account an individual's unique dietary needs and

preferences. For example, a food sensor may not be able to distinguish between two similar foods that have different nutritional profiles. Additionally, a food sensor may not be able to provide information about the taste or texture of a food, which can be important factors in making dietary choices.

In conclusion, while food sensors can be a valuable tool for monitoring food intake and making healthier choices, they are not without their drawbacks. People should carefully consider the potential limitations of food sensors before investing in them and should use them in moderation as part of a balanced approach to healthy eating.

## Real-world examples of using food sensors for healthy eating

Food sensors are an emerging technology that can help people make more informed choices about the food they eat. There are already several real-world examples of food sensors being used for healthy eating.

1. SCiO

SCiO is a handheld device that uses near-infrared spectroscopy to analyze the molecular composition of food. Users can simply scan their food with the device and get an instant analysis of its nutritional content. The device can identify the amounts of fat, protein, carbohydrates, and other nutrients in a given food item. This can be useful for people who are tracking their nutrient intake, such as athletes and people with specific dietary needs.

2. NutriRay3D

NutriRay3D is a food scanner that uses 3D imaging to analyze the shape and volume of food items. The device can then estimate the number of calories in the food based on its shape and volume. The NutriRay3D can be used to scan whole meals, allowing users to get a more accurate picture of their overall calorie intake.

3. HAPIfork

HAPIfork is a smart fork that helps users eat more slowly and mindfully. The fork vibrates when the user eats too quickly, reminding them to slow down. The fork also tracks how quickly the user is eating and provides data on their eating habits over time. Eating more slowly can help people feel fuller and more satisfied with their meals, leading to fewer calories consumed overall.

4. TellSpec

TellSpec is a handheld device that uses spectrometry to analyze the chemical composition of food. Users can scan their food with the device and get a breakdown of its nutritional content, including calories, fat, protein, and carbohydrates. TellSpec can also detect the presence of allergens and other harmful substances in food, making it a useful tool for people with food sensitivities.

5. SmartPlate

SmartPlate is a plate that uses image recognition to analyze the nutritional content of a meal. Users can take a picture of their food with their smartphone and upload it to the SmartPlate app. The app then provides a breakdown of the meal's nutritional content, including calories, fat, protein, and carbohydrates. SmartPlate can also provide suggestions for healthier alternatives to the foods the user is eating.

Overall, food sensors are a promising technology that can help people make more informed choices about the food they eat. While they are not without their limitations, real-world examples of food sensors being used for healthy eating suggest that they have the potential to improve dietary habits and promote healthier lifestyles.

## Chapter 6: Comparing and Combining Methods
## Side-by-side comparison of the five methods for optimizing and monitoring eating habits

In the world of healthy eating, there are various methods and technologies available to help individuals monitor and optimize their eating habits. In this chapter, we will compare and contrast the five primary methods discussed in the previous chapters: DNA Nudge, food tracking apps, smart kitchen appliances, nutritional coaching, and food sensors.

To begin with, let's summarize the key features of each method:

- DNA Nudge: uses genetic information to provide personalized food recommendations and limit unhealthy choices at the point of sale.

- Food tracking apps: allow users to log their food intake and monitor their progress towards health goals.

- Smart kitchen appliances: utilize technology such as Bluetooth and Wi-Fi to enhance cooking and meal preparation, such as precision cooking and recipe suggestions.

- Nutritional coaching: involves one-on-one or group sessions with a qualified coach to provide education, support, and accountability for healthy eating habits.

- Food sensors: can be used to scan food products and provide real-time nutritional information, including allergen warnings and ingredient lists.

Now, let's dive into the side-by-side comparison of each method based on several key factors.

Accuracy and Personalization DNA Nudge is one of the most personalized methods due to the use of genetic data to provide recommendations. The food tracking apps and nutritional coaching can also be personalized based on the individual's preferences and goals. Food sensors provide accurate nutritional information based on the product scanned, but they are not personalized to the individual's needs. Smart kitchen appliances offer precision cooking and recipe suggestions, but they do not provide personalized nutritional information.

Ease of Use and Accessibility Food tracking apps and smart kitchen appliances are user-friendly and accessible to anyone with a smartphone or a compatible device. DNA Nudge requires a genetic test and the use of a wearable device, while nutritional coaching may require scheduling appointments and travel. Food sensors may be less accessible and not widely available in all regions.

Cost The cost of each method varies. DNA Nudge requires a one-time genetic test and the purchase of a wearable device. Food tracking apps and some smart kitchen appliances are often free or available at a low cost. Nutritional coaching typically involves ongoing sessions with a qualified coach, which can be costly. Food sensors can be expensive and require frequent purchases to maintain their use.

Effectiveness and Long-Term Sustainability All methods have demonstrated some level of effectiveness in improving healthy eating habits. DNA Nudge has shown promising results in reducing consumption of unhealthy foods and increasing nutrient intake. Food tracking apps have been effective in promoting healthy eating habits and weight loss. Smart kitchen appliances can help individuals cook healthy meals at home and decrease reliance on unhealthy processed foods. Nutritional coaching provides personalized support and accountability, which can be effective for individuals who need guidance in making healthy choices. Food sensors can be effective in identifying allergens and hidden ingredients, but may not provide long-term behavioral change.

Overall, each method has its strengths and weaknesses. DNA Nudge, food tracking apps, and smart kitchen appliances offer a high level of personalization and ease of use, but may require an upfront investment.

Nutritional coaching provides personalized support and accountability, but may be costly and require ongoing sessions. Food sensors can provide accurate information but may not offer a long-term solution for healthy eating habits.

Combining methods can be an effective way to maximize the benefits of each approach. For example, using a food tracking app in conjunction with a smart kitchen appliance and nutritional coaching can provide a well-rounded approach to monitoring and optimizing healthy eating habits.

In conclusion, selecting the right method or combination of methods to optimize and monitor eating habits depends on individual preferences, needs, and goals. Understanding the strengths and limitations of each method can help individuals make an informed decision and select the best approach for their personal situation.

| Method | Key Features | Key Factors Compared |
|---|---|---|
| DNA Nudge | Genetic testing to provide personalized dietary recommendations, immediate feedback at point of purchase | Accuracy of genetic testing, cost, accessibility, ease of use, potential privacy concerns |
| Food Tracking Apps | Allows for tracking of food intake, provides nutritional information, and analysis of eating habits over time | Accuracy of food tracking, ease of use, availability of features, compatibility with other apps and devices, potential for obsessive behavior |
| Smart Kitchen Appliances | Use of technology such as smart scales and cooking devices to help with portion control and healthier cooking techniques | Cost, ease of use, integration with other devices, potential for reliance on technology |
| Nutritional Coaching | One-on-one coaching with a certified nutritionist to provide personalized recommendations and support | Qualifications of coach, cost, accessibility, personalized support, potential for conflicting advice |
| Food Sensors | Use of devices to measure nutrient levels in food or monitor consumption of certain nutrients | Accuracy of sensors, ease of use, compatibility with other devices, cost, potential for overreliance on technology |

The table can be customized to include other factors that may be relevant to the reader.

## Tips for combining methods

Combining multiple methods for optimizing and monitoring eating habits can be an effective way to achieve a balanced and healthy diet. While each method has its own unique advantages and drawbacks, combining them can address these limitations and provide a more comprehensive approach to healthy eating.

Here are some tips for combining methods:

1. Start with your goals: Before combining methods, it's important to identify your goals and what you hope to achieve. For example, if your goal is to lose weight, you may want to focus on tracking your food intake and using a DNA test to identify foods that are best for your body. If your goal is to improve your overall health, you may want to combine nutritional coaching with the use of smart kitchen appliances to prepare healthier meals.

2. Identify complementary methods: Look for methods that complement each other and address different aspects of healthy eating. For example, combining food tracking apps with smart kitchen appliances can help you track your food intake and prepare healthy meals at home. DNA testing can provide insights into your body's response to certain foods and help you make more informed decisions about what to eat. Nutritional coaching can provide

personalized guidance on healthy eating habits and help you set and achieve goals.

3. Start small: Combining multiple methods can be overwhelming, so start with one or two methods and gradually incorporate others over time. For example, start by using a food tracking app to monitor your food intake and gradually introduce a smart kitchen appliance to prepare healthier meals.

4. Use technology to your advantage: Many of these methods rely on technology, so make sure you're using it to your advantage. Use apps and other tools to track your progress, set reminders, and stay motivated. Consider using a wearable device to track your physical activity and monitor your sleep patterns.

5. Be flexible: Combining multiple methods requires flexibility and the ability to adapt to changing circumstances. For example, if you're traveling or eating out, you may need to rely more heavily on food tracking apps and nutritional coaching to make healthy choices.

6. Keep track of your progress: It's important to monitor your progress and adjust your approach as needed. Use the data from food tracking apps and other methods to identify patterns and make adjustments to your diet and lifestyle.

By combining multiple methods, you can take a more comprehensive approach to healthy eating and increase your chances of success. Just remember to start small, identify complementary methods, use technology to your advantage, and stay flexible and adaptable as you work towards your goals.

| Goal | Methods to Combine |
| --- | --- |
| Increase nutrient intake | Use food tracking app to monitor nutrients, use smart kitchen appliances to prepare nutrient-rich meals, work with nutritional coach to optimize nutrient balance |
| Decrease calorie intake | Use food tracking app to monitor calories, use DNA Nudge to receive personalized food recommendations, use food sensor to monitor calorie intake |
| Reduce food waste | Use smart kitchen appliances to repurpose leftovers, use food tracking app to plan meals and shop more efficiently |
| Improve digestion | Use food tracking app to monitor trigger foods, work with nutritional coach to identify and address digestive issues, use smart kitchen appliances to prepare digestion-friendly meals |
| Optimize athletic performance | Use DNA Nudge to receive personalized food and hydration recommendations, work with nutritional coach to develop a performance-optimized diet, use food tracking app to monitor nutrient intake |

Note that these combinations are just examples and may not be suitable for everyone. It's important to consult with a healthcare professional or registered dietitian to create a personalized plan for your specific needs and goals.

# Real-world examples of using multiple methods for healthy eating" the sub topic for about 3000 words long

Combining different methods for healthy eating can be a powerful approach to achieving your dietary goals. While each method has its own advantages and disadvantages, using them together can provide a more comprehensive picture of your diet and lifestyle. Here are some real-world examples of how combining different methods has helped individuals improve their eating habits.

1. Using food tracking apps with nutritional coaching One effective way to use food tracking apps is in conjunction with nutritional coaching. While the app can help you monitor your food intake and identify areas for improvement, a coach can provide personalized advice and support to help you achieve your goals. For example, a coach can help you identify the right macronutrient balance for your body type, provide guidance on how to eat for specific health conditions, and offer strategies for dealing with emotional eating. Combining the two methods can help you stay accountable and make lasting changes to your diet.

2. Using smart kitchen appliances with meal planning Smart kitchen appliances, such as a smart scale or blender, can make meal preparation and portion control easier. But to

maximize their effectiveness, it's important to combine them with meal planning. By planning your meals in advance, you can ensure that you have the right ingredients on hand, reduce food waste, and make healthy choices more consistently. You can also use your smart kitchen appliances to batch-cook healthy meals, which can save you time and ensure that you always have a nutritious meal available.

3. Using food sensors with personalized nutrition advice Food sensors can provide valuable information about the quality and nutrient content of your food. By using a food sensor, you can get a more accurate picture of the calories, macronutrients, and micronutrients in your meals. To get the most out of this method, it's important to combine it with personalized nutrition advice. A qualified nutritionist can help you interpret the data from your food sensor, and provide guidance on how to make healthy adjustments to your diet. For example, if your food sensor indicates that you're not getting enough protein, a nutritionist can suggest high-protein foods to add to your diet.

4. Using nutritional coaching with a support group Nutritional coaching can be a valuable tool for improving your eating habits, but it can also be helpful to have a support group. A support group can provide motivation, accountability, and camaraderie as you work to achieve your

goals. For example, you might join a group of like-minded individuals who are also trying to eat healthier, or you might work with a coach who also leads a support group. By combining the two methods, you can benefit from both individualized support and group encouragement.

5. Using food tracking apps with smart kitchen appliances Using food tracking apps in conjunction with smart kitchen appliances can help you optimize your eating habits. For example, you can use your food tracking app to monitor your intake of specific macronutrients, such as protein or carbs, and adjust your meal plan accordingly. You can then use your smart kitchen appliances to prepare and measure your meals precisely, ensuring that you're getting the right amount of each nutrient. This combination can be particularly effective for individuals with specific dietary goals, such as athletes or people with certain medical conditions.

In conclusion, combining different methods can be an effective way to optimize your eating habits. By using multiple tools and strategies, you can get a more complete picture of your diet, make healthy choices more consistently, and achieve your goals more effectively.

## Choosing the best methods for your individual needs and preferences

Choosing the best methods for optimizing and monitoring eating habits is a highly individualized process. What works for one person may not work for another. Therefore, it is essential to consider one's personal needs and preferences when selecting the most appropriate method or combination of methods.

Here are some factors to consider when choosing the best methods for your individual needs and preferences:

1. Goals: What are your specific health goals? For example, if your primary goal is weight loss, then you may want to consider using a food tracking app, smart kitchen appliances, and nutritional coaching to help you achieve your desired weight.

2. Lifestyle: What is your lifestyle like? Do you have a busy schedule that requires quick and easy meal options? If so, then you may want to consider using smart kitchen appliances or food delivery services to make meal prep more manageable.

3. Budget: What is your budget? Some methods, such as nutritional coaching, can be expensive, while others, such as food tracking apps, are relatively inexpensive. Consider what you are willing and able to spend to achieve your goals.

4. Personal preferences: What types of foods do you enjoy eating? What types of exercise do you enjoy doing? Consider your personal preferences when selecting a method or combination of methods that will work best for you.

5. Health conditions: Do you have any health conditions that require specific dietary needs? If so, then you may want to consider working with a nutritional coach who specializes in your specific health condition.

Once you have considered these factors, it is time to select the best methods or combination of methods for your individual needs and preferences. Here are some examples of how you might choose the best methods for your individual needs and preferences:

Example 1: Sarah's goal is to lose weight, and she has a busy schedule. She decides to use a food tracking app to monitor her caloric intake and a smart kitchen appliance to make meal prep easier. She also decides to sign up for a meal delivery service to save time and help her stay on track with her weight loss goals.

Example 2: John has diabetes and needs to monitor his blood sugar levels closely. He decides to work with a nutritional coach who specializes in diabetes management to help him make dietary changes to manage his condition. He also uses a food tracking app to monitor his daily intake of carbohydrates and other nutrients.

Example 3: Emily loves to cook and wants to learn new recipes that are healthy and delicious. She decides to work with a nutritional coach who specializes in recipe development to help her learn new cooking techniques and meal ideas. She also uses a food tracking app to monitor her nutrient intake and a food sensor to help her measure the nutrient content of her meals.

In conclusion, choosing the best methods for optimizing and monitoring eating habits requires consideration of one's personal needs and preferences. By taking into account one's goals, lifestyle, budget, personal preferences, and health conditions, individuals can select the best methods or combination of methods that will work best for them.

## Conclusion

## Summary of the book's main points

In this book, we have explored various methods for optimizing and monitoring eating habits, with the ultimate goal of promoting healthy eating and improving overall well-being. Each of the five methods - meal planning, food tracking apps, smart kitchen appliances, nutritional coaching, and food sensors - has its own unique advantages and drawbacks. However, by combining these methods and utilizing their strengths, individuals can create a personalized approach to healthy eating that works for them.

The first method, meal planning, is an effective way to take control of one's diet by pre-planning meals and snacks. By creating a grocery list and shopping with intention, individuals can ensure that their meals are well-balanced and nutritious. Meal planning can also save time and money by reducing food waste and limiting the need for last-minute takeout or fast food options.

Food tracking apps are another valuable tool for promoting healthy eating. By logging food and beverage intake, individuals can gain insight into their eating habits, track progress towards goals, and identify areas for improvement. Food tracking apps also provide access to nutritional information and can help individuals make informed choices when dining out or grocery shopping.

Smart kitchen appliances, such as air fryers and smart scales, offer convenience and versatility in the kitchen while promoting healthy eating habits. These appliances can help individuals cook meals quickly and efficiently while limiting the use of unhealthy cooking methods like deep-frying. Smart kitchen appliances can also aid in portion control by accurately measuring ingredients and helping individuals avoid overeating.

Nutritional coaching is a valuable resource for individuals looking to develop a personalized approach to healthy eating. A qualified nutritional coach can provide guidance and support, help individuals set and achieve goals, and offer accountability and motivation. Nutritional coaching can also help individuals navigate complex dietary restrictions or health conditions.

Finally, food sensors are an emerging technology that can help individuals monitor their food intake and promote healthy eating habits. These sensors can provide real-time data on nutrient intake, meal frequency, and eating patterns, which can help individuals make more informed food choices and identify areas for improvement.

While each of these methods has its own strengths and limitations, combining them can create a comprehensive approach to healthy eating that is tailored to individual needs and preferences. For example, an individual might use meal planning and smart kitchen appliances to prepare healthy meals at home, while using food tracking apps to monitor their food intake throughout the day. Additionally, nutritional coaching can provide support and guidance throughout the process, and food sensors can provide additional insight into eating patterns and nutrient intake.

Ultimately, the key to choosing the best methods for promoting healthy eating is understanding one's own needs and preferences. By taking a personalized approach and combining methods to suit individual goals, individuals can achieve long-term success in improving their eating habits and overall well-being.

# Final thoughts on optimizing and monitoring eating habits

As we come to the end of this book on optimizing and monitoring eating habits, it is important to reflect on some final thoughts that can help us in our journey towards healthier and more mindful eating habits. While the methods we have explored in this book are diverse, they all share a common goal: to help us make more informed choices about what we eat and how we eat it. Here are some final thoughts on how to best achieve that goal.

1. No one method is a silver bullet

As we have seen throughout this book, each of the methods we explored has its strengths and limitations. While some may work better for some individuals than others, it is important to remember that no one method is a silver bullet. Rather, the most effective approach is likely to involve a combination of methods that work best for our individual needs and preferences.

1. Mindfulness is key

No matter which methods we choose to adopt, the most important factor in optimizing and monitoring our eating habits is mindfulness. By being present and fully engaged in the act of eating, we can better understand our relationship with food and make more informed choices about what we put in our bodies.

2. Be patient and kind to yourself

Changing our eating habits can be a challenging process, and it is important to remember that it is a journey, not a destination. Rather than expecting instant results or becoming discouraged by setbacks, we should focus on making small, sustainable changes over time. And just as importantly, we should be kind and patient with ourselves throughout the process.

3. Seek support when needed

While adopting healthy eating habits is a personal journey, we do not have to do it alone. Seeking support from friends, family, or professionals like nutritionists or counselors can help us stay motivated and on track.

4. Remember the big picture

As we focus on optimizing and monitoring our eating habits, it is important to keep in mind the big picture. Eating well is just one part of a healthy lifestyle, which also includes regular exercise, sufficient sleep, and stress management. By taking a holistic approach to our health, we can achieve the greatest long-term benefits.

In conclusion, optimizing and monitoring our eating habits is an ongoing journey that requires patience, mindfulness, and a willingness to try new methods. By taking a personalized, multifaceted approach that incorporates the methods we have explored in this book, we can develop a healthier, more balanced relationship with food that supports our overall health and well-being.

## Call to action for readers to take control of their health through healthy eating habits

Healthy eating habits are vital for maintaining good health and preventing chronic diseases. In the previous chapters, we have explored various methods and technologies that can help individuals optimize and monitor their eating habits. These methods and technologies include nutritional tracking apps, smart kitchen appliances, nutritional coaching, food sensors, and combining multiple methods.

While these tools can be incredibly helpful, they are only effective if they are used consistently and with purpose. The reality is that creating and maintaining healthy eating habits is a long-term commitment that requires motivation and dedication. In this final section, we will provide a call to action for readers to take control of their health through healthy eating habits.

The first step to taking control of your health through healthy eating habits is to acknowledge that change is necessary. Often, people find it challenging to make changes to their eating habits, especially if they have been following a particular routine for an extended period. However, with the right mindset, positive attitude, and consistent effort, change is possible.

Once you have made the decision to change, the next step is to set specific, measurable, and achievable goals. These goals should be tailored to your individual needs and preferences. For example, you might aim to reduce your daily sugar intake, increase your vegetable consumption, or drink more water. By setting achievable goals, you will have a clear plan of action and can track your progress over time.

The third step is to take advantage of the tools and technologies that we have discussed in this book. By incorporating nutritional tracking apps, smart kitchen appliances, nutritional coaching, and food sensors, you will have a clear understanding of your eating habits and can make adjustments as necessary. By combining multiple methods, you can gain a comprehensive view of your eating habits and can take a more holistic approach to improving your health.

Another important aspect of healthy eating habits is to focus on whole, nutrient-dense foods. These foods, such as fruits, vegetables, whole grains, and lean proteins, are packed with essential vitamins, minerals, and nutrients that are vital for optimal health. By focusing on whole foods and avoiding highly processed foods, you can reduce your risk of chronic diseases and maintain a healthy weight.

In addition to focusing on whole foods, it is important to practice mindful eating. Mindful eating is a practice that involves paying attention to the present moment, savoring the flavors and textures of the food, and listening to your body's hunger and fullness cues. By practicing mindful eating, you can cultivate a more positive relationship with food and make more intentional choices that support your health and well-being.

In conclusion, optimizing and monitoring your eating habits is crucial for maintaining good health and preventing chronic diseases. By taking advantage of the tools and technologies that we have discussed, setting achievable goals, focusing on whole, nutrient-dense foods, and practicing mindful eating, you can take control of your health and make long-lasting changes that will benefit you for years to come. Remember, change is possible, and by taking action today, you can create a healthier and happier future for yourself.

**THE END**

# Potential References

Introduction:

Mozaffarian, D. (2016). Dietary and policy priorities for cardiovascular disease, diabetes, and obesity: a comprehensive review. Circulation, 133(2), 187-225.

Fenech, M. (2018). Nutriepigenomics and its implications for health. International Journal of Molecular Sciences, 19(12), 4103.

DeBusk, R., & Jablonski, K. (2019). Precision nutrition: A new approach to improving health. American Journal of Lifestyle Medicine, 13(4), 348-351.

Chapter 1: DNA Nudge

Celis-Morales, C., Livingstone, K. M., Marsaux, C. F. M., Macready, A. L., Fallaize, R., O'Donovan, C. B., ... & Mathers, J. C. (2017). Effect of personalized nutrition on health-related behaviour change: evidence from the Food4me European randomized controlled trial. International Journal of Epidemiology, 46(2), 578-588.

Nielsen, D. E., El-Sohemy, A., & Underhill, T. M. (2017). Nutrigenetics and nutrigenomics insights into dietary strategies to improve lipid metabolism: a systematic review. Journal of Lipid Research, 58(11), 2239-2254.

Chapter 2: Food Tracking Apps

Burke, L. E., Wang, J., & Sevick, M. A. (2011). Self-monitoring in weight loss: a systematic review of the literature. Journal of the American Dietetic Association, 111(1), 92-102.

Green, J., & Hargreaves, J. (2019). Disclosing app data sharing to consumers. Nature Human Behaviour, 3(11), 1179-1183.

## Chapter 3: Smart Kitchen Appliances

Micucci, D., Mencarini, E., Valentini, M., & Frontoni, E. (2018). Vision-based smart kitchen for supporting healthy lifestyle. Journal of Ambient Intelligence and Humanized Computing, 9(5), 1411-1424.

Kanjo, E., & Al-Husseini, L. (2018). Smart kitchen: IoT sensing for better food management. IEEE Pervasive Computing, 17(1), 39-47.

## Chapter 4: Nutritional Coaching

Colby, S., Johnson, M. R., Lucas, H., & Stringer, C. (2020). "Nutrition coaching improves health outcomes: A systematic review to assess the impact of nutrition coaching on metabolic syndrome parameters." Journal of the Academy of Nutrition and Dietetics, 120(4), 669-679.

Minter, C., & Thomas, J. G. (2018). "Nutritional counseling in primary care: A systematic review of current practice."

Journal of the American Association of Nurse Practitioners, 30(8), 455-462.

Morgan, P. J., Collins, C. E., Plotnikoff, R. C., Callister, R., Burrows, T., Fletcher, R., ... & Young, M. D. (2019). "The SHED-IT community trial study protocol: a randomised controlled trial of weight-loss programs for overweight and obese men." International Journal of Behavioral Nutrition and Physical Activity, 16(1), 46.

Chapter 5: Food Sensors

Oliver, J. E., Shastri, A., & Bari, M. F. (2020). Advances in Food Quality Monitoring: A Comprehensive Review of Modern and Emerging Food Sensor Technologies. Foods, 9(11), 1604.

Maksimainen, J., Salmela, L., Hokkanen, J., & Lilleberg, L. (2019). Smart sensors and their applications for food quality and safety. Journal of Food Engineering, 262, 1-10.

Chapter 6: Comparing and Combining Methods

Willems, M., Claassen, G. D., van der Wielen, N., & Kremer, S. (2019). A comparative study on the usability of five different nutrition applications. Nutrients, 11(6), 1286.

Wang, D., Wu, L., & Lu, Y. (2020). Personalized nutrition service platform design based on food classification and clustering. Future Generation Computer Systems, 109, 68-80.

Conclusion:

Schor, J. (2019). Using Nutrigenomics to Personalize Diets. IEEE Pulse, 10(5), 39-43.

Vogt, N., Taff, E., & Kretser, A. (2019). Assessing the impact of mobile applications on health and wellness. Journal of Medical Systems, 43(5), 108.

www.ingramcontent.com/pod-product-compliance
Lightning Source LLC
LaVergne TN
LVHW010411070526
838199LV00065B/5945